A Trip To The Seaside

The day was finally here! We had been looking forward to it all summer - our family trip to the seaside! We woke up early that morning, eager to get the day started.

It was a bright and promising sunny morning. We checked the weather forecast and it was set to be a glorious day.

Everybody was in an excited rush to get ready.

In the kitchen a mountain of bread was being buttered for sandwiches, and in the rest of the house everybody scrambled around trying to find bathing suits.

We packed the car to the brim with everything that we would need for the day: towels, sunglasses, sun hats, chairs, and a large picnic with lots of cool drinks.

And before I knew it, we were on the way! As we hit the road we listened to our favourite songs by The Beatles. We all began singing "Yellow Submarine" at the top of our voices together, laughing at how badly out of tune we were.

After an hour or so of driving I began to see the glimmering ocean in the distance. I could feel the salty breeze coming through the car windows.

I put my hand out and felt the wind blowing through my fingers. In the distance I could see the water, vast and glistening in the morning sun.

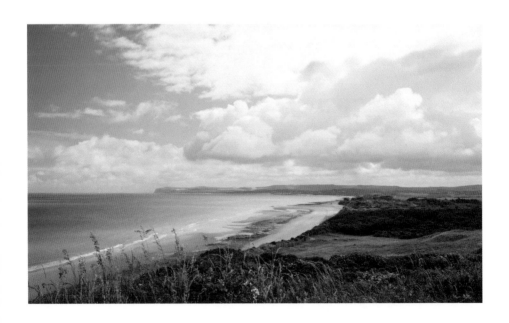

As we arrived into the seaside town we drove down the narrow streets to try to find a parking space. The town was picture perfect.

Each road was lined with colourful shops and cafes, with tourists happily strolling around enjoying ice creams. The air was filled with the sound of laughter and music.

I could smell the delicious, unmistakeable scent of fish and chips wafting through the air.

We found a parking space a few minutes walk from the beach.

As we wandered down the cobbled street I took in the sights. On the corner was a charming local pub with people sat outside enjoying food and drinks in the sun. A man walked past with his dog, it's tail wagging happily behind.

Further down the road was a small antique shop selling treasures from the past. From a quick glance I could see that the goods on display were all coastal themed: delicate models of sailboats and lighthouses, and nautical instruments that looked like they had come straight off a ship.

I must come back to this shop, I thought.

Moving on from the beautiful shop display window, we crossed the road and reached the beach. We all stopped and took in the view: it was breathtaking.

There was nothing but a blue expanse of water for as far as the eye could see.

Smiling happily at each other, we made our way onto the beach. We began to laugh as sand quickly made its way into our shoes, so we took them off and walked barefoot instead.

How warm the sand felt beneath our feet!

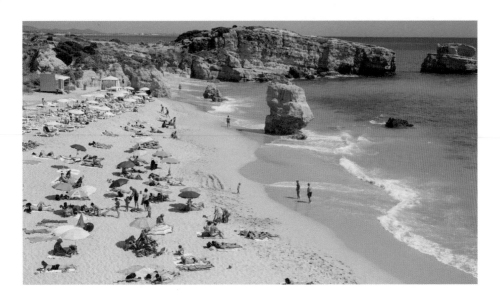

It had been so long since I last visited a beach, I had forgotten the velvety smooth feel of sand. It was like a fine powder, so soft to touch.

After wandering around for a few minutes we found the perfect spot to set up. We spread out our towels and sat down. It was a beautiful sight, seeing the ocean glinting in the light.

The sound of children's laughter filled the air as they splashed in the waves and built sandcastles.

The air was filled with the sweet scent of salt and seaweed.

The sun was high in the sky, with not a cloud in sight, and the ocean waves gently rolled in and out.

Stroll Along The Beach

I decided to go for a walk along the shore. It had been so long since I had dipped my feet in the ocean. It was gloriously cool and refreshing.

I felt so relaxed, feeling the soft wet sand between my toes and the waves lapping at my ankles. Nothing else mattered in the world right now, I was completely at peace.

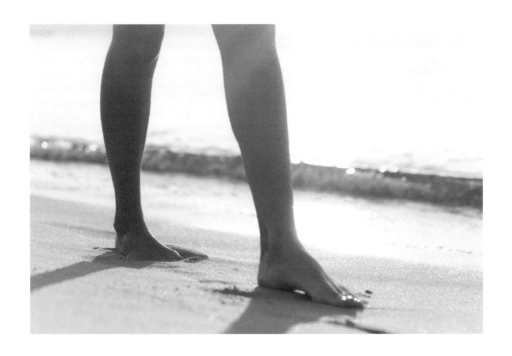

The water was a beautiful shade of blue-green, with the sunlight reflecting off the waves.

The sand was soft and white, with small shells and pebbles scattered along the shore.

I remembered learning in school about how seashells were formed.

Shells are made by molluscs, such as clams, scallops, mussels and oysters. When a mollusc is hatched from an egg it begins to build its outer shell, layer by layer. As the mollusc grows in size, they enlarge their shell to fit their growing body.

I picked a shell up. It was a strange shape, yet it fitted nicely in my hand. It felt cool to the touch.

I ran my finger over its smooth bumps and traced the spiralled pattern.

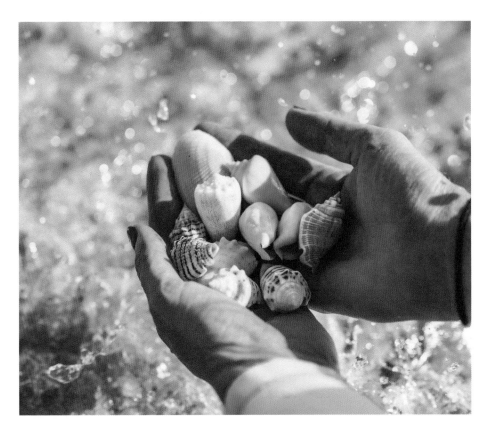

It was pearl white in colour, with pink and purple swirls. I had never seen a shell like this before.

I held it up to my ear and heard the whooshing sound of the ocean. Back and forth, in and out.

It was a gentle, soothing noise. A continuous, relaxing rhythm.

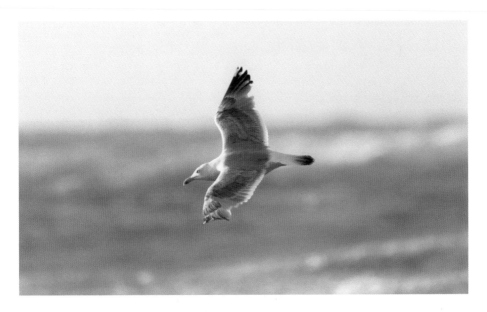

I watched as seagulls flew overhead, their wings flapping gracefully in the air.

I watched them for a few moments, wondering what it would feel like to soar above the ocean like they did.

They glided effortlessly through the air, their movements fluid and graceful. How it must feel to be weightless, and to fly wherever you want.

As I continued walking, I saw a family playing in the sand, building sandcastles and laughing with each other. I smiled at them as I walked past, and they smiled back.

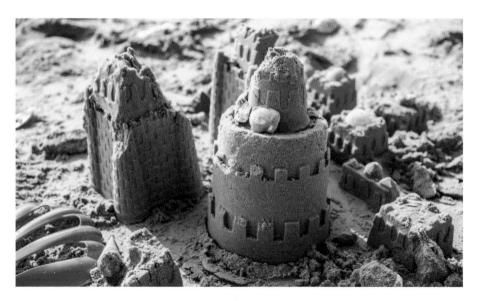

The Cave

I reached a rocky area of the shore and began to explore. Taking my time and stepping carefully, I moved along the rocks. There were so many nooks and crannies!

Some rocks were completely covered in seaweed and barnacles, with small pools of warm water in between them. Tiny fish darted around in the water, and small crabs scuttled along the rocks edge.

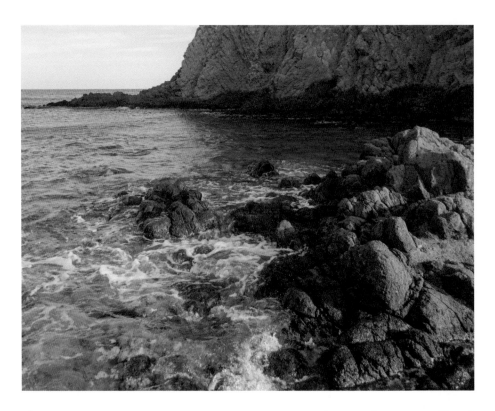

I saw a small cave up ahead, nestled within the rocks. I carried on climbing along, enjoying the adventure.

I was using my hands and feet now to go along the rocks, moving slowly to reach the entrance of the cave.

The cave was cool and damp, and the sound of the waves echoed within its walls. It was incredible. I felt like I had uncovered a secret hideaway, a part of the beach that was all mine.

How long had this cave existed for, I wondered. And who else had discovered it in the past? Was I the first?

As I moved further into the hollow cave the ocean water was more gentle. The walls of the cave seemed to sparkle, like glittering crystals. The water reflected the sunlight, bringing a dazzling display of shimmering light.

The whole place seemed to have a magical glow to it.

Small stalactites hung from the ceiling of the cave. Some were thin like icicles, and some were chunky like ice cream cones. As I stared up at them, admiring their jagged pointy tips, a drop of water fell off one and splashed onto my nose. I chuckled to myself.

The sounds from the beach seemed more distant now. Time seemed to stand still in this special cavern, this hidden world of beauty and wonder.

I felt a great sense of peace and tranquility wash over me. I felt like I could stay there forever, just floating in the gentle waves and listening to the sound of my own breath.

After enjoying the peacefulness of the cave for a while I decided to make my way back to my family on the beach. My stomach was beginning to rumble and I couldn't wait to have a sip of ice cold juice from our cooler bag.

I strolled back along the sand. The beach was alive with activity, as people swam, sunbathed and played games.

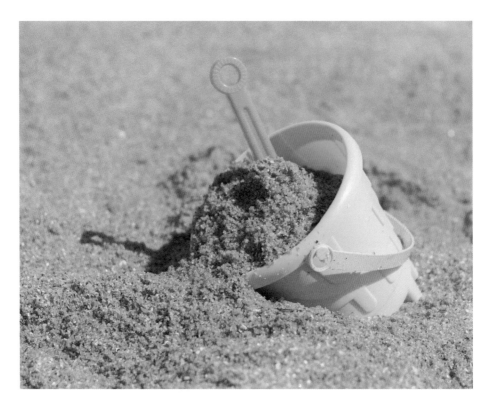

I saw a Dad and his son playing with a bat and ball together. They were having so much fun, laughing and running around.

It was midday and more people had arrived at the beach now. There was a busy and fun atmosphere.

I heard happy laughter come from a family nearby. The children were building a moat with their parents, taking it in turns to collect water with their buckets. In the middle of the moat was a huge sandcastle decorated with pebbles and shells.

Further on, I heard cheers come from a group of boys and girls. They were kicking a football and somebody had just scored. Their goal area was made from piles of seaweed, which made me chuckle.

After a short walk I reached my family and told them all about my adventure with the rocky cave as we unpacked our picnic.

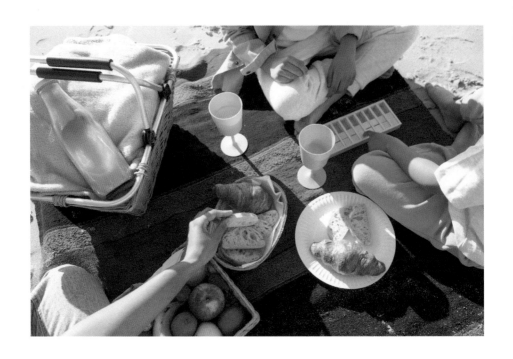

We sat down on our beach chairs and began to tuck in to the food.

I had made my favourite sandwiches for lunch - ham and cheese. Everyone else shared pork pies, chicken salad, and sausage rolls.

It was a lovely feeling, sharing this happy moment with my family and watching the world go by.

We chatted and laughed together, enjoying the sounds of the busy beach around us.

The Antique Shop

After lunch, I decided to take a stroll back to the antiques shop we had passed earlier. I had always been fascinated by antiques - unique objects that came with their own story and history. The sign above the shop door looked like an antique in itself. It was a large wooden sign with fading blue and white paint.

'Sailor's Trove' it read.

I opened the door and stepped inside. The interior of the shop was dimly lit, but the sunlight filtered through the windows, casting a soft glow on the objects displayed on the shelves.

I could smell polished wood and sea salt in the air. It was quiet in the shop, with only the gentle sound of a ticking grandfather clock.

There were so many treasures on display: antique compasses, hand drawn world maps, brass telescopes and large seashells.

I marvelled at the delicate models of ships, so much care and attention had been put into these beautiful pieces.

As I browsed the shelves I was approached by an elderly man with a kind smile. He introduced himself as the owner and told me this had been his shop for sixty years. It was a family business that had passed through the generations, and he began working there when he was a teenager with his father.

When the shop had first opened many years ago, the seaside town had been a bustling port for ships carrying goods from all over the world. Sailors would visit the town to trade their wares, and the shop had been a popular destination for sailors looking for unique souvenirs to bring back to their families. I was fascinated listening to the owner's stories of the history of the town.

On one of the shelves rested an antique officer's spyglass. It was a fine piece, with its polished mahogany body and brass tube.

I picked it up, extending it to its full length and peered through the eyepiece.

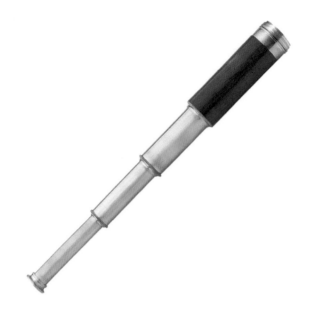

For such an old instrument I was amazed at how clear and strong the magnification was.

I looked out of the shop window, adjusting the spyglass. I could see far out to sea, spotting a small fishing boat in the distance.

The shop owner told me the spyglass had been used by sailors and captains at sea, to look out for enemy ships on the horizon, or to find land. They were also known as naval or nautical telescopes. With the help of compasses, many sailors would use spyglasses to observe the stars, to help direct them on the open sea.

I gently placed the spyglass back on the shelf and asked the owner what other unique treasures he had in his shop.

With a smile, he reached for a small leather-bound journal which was tucked away on a shelf. He gave it to me.

The leather was a deep, rich brown colour, and soft to the touch. The book had clearly seen it's fair share of adventure. The binding and edges were frayed from years of handling.

I opened it, and saw that it was filled with hand written notes and sketches, documenting a sailor's journey across the seas.

The pages inside revealed intricate drawings of landscapes and ports. On one page was a detailed drawing of a man with curly hair, sat on a bench with a large shaggy dog at his side.

The owner smiled and told me the drawing was of his grandfather, who had been a sailor. This diary had belonged to him.

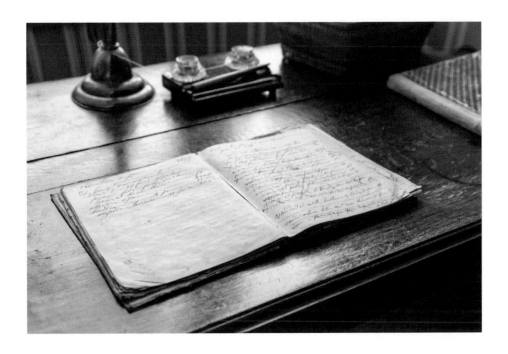

His grandfather had travelled the world, reaching faraway lands to trade tea and exotic spices.

As he journeyed across the sea, he documented his adventures in the journal, sketching the landscapes and people he met along the way.

I pored over the pages, lapping up the details. I felt like I had been transported to a different time and place. Although the ink had begun to fade over the years, the attention to detail was incredible.

I gently turned the page and saw a detailed drawing of a lighthouse, standing tall and proud on a bed of rocks.

The lighthouse was surrounded by crashing waves, with the sun setting in the background. It was a beautiful drawing.

"Have you visited the lighthouse yet?" asked the owner, "it has been the focal point of our town for several hundred years."

I told him I hadn't.

"You must go" he said, "it is incredibly beautiful."

The Lighthouse

As I walked down the cobbled streets, following the shop owners directions to the lighthouse, I marvelled at what an incredible day it had been so far. This small seaside town had so much to offer, and so much history.

As I strolled along, enjoying the warmth of the sun, I saw an ice cream parlour.
I couldn't resist.

I left the shop a few minutes later with a mint choc chip ice cream cone, delicious! I loved ice cream, especially on days as hot as today.

Slurping away at my ice cream, catching any drips as they melted in the sun, I continued down the road and reached the promenade.

I could see the lighthouse a short way ahead. Its tall, white structure stood out against the endless blue of the sea and sky.

The promenade was bustling with activity, with children running around and laughing, and couples strolling hand in hand.

I could hear music playing from somewhere too, it sounded like a brass band. It was a lively and cheerful atmosphere, and I felt myself smiling from the joy and excitement of it all.

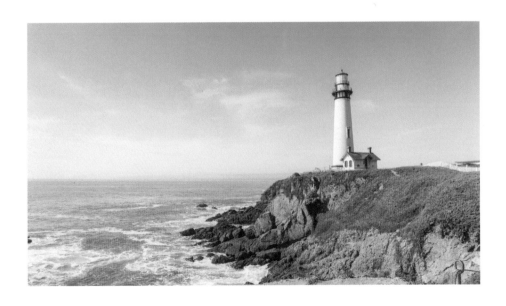

The lighthouse was taller than I expected, and even more striking than the drawing I had seen of it.

At the base of the lighthouse the ocean waves crashed against the rocks, each one more powerful than the last. The frothing white water foamed into spirals, creating intricate patterns on the waves. The midday sun shone high in the sky, and the water seemed to dance with every ripple and movement.

I reached the entrance of the lighthouse and ran my hands over the rough stonework.

Although it was clearly an old building that had seen its fair share of stormy weather over the years, it was in very good condition. I began to climb the stairs, hearing the seagulls flying overhead, squabbling with each other.

The steps were painted yellow and worn from so many people walking up them. After what felt like hundreds of steps, I finally reached the top.

The view was spectacular.

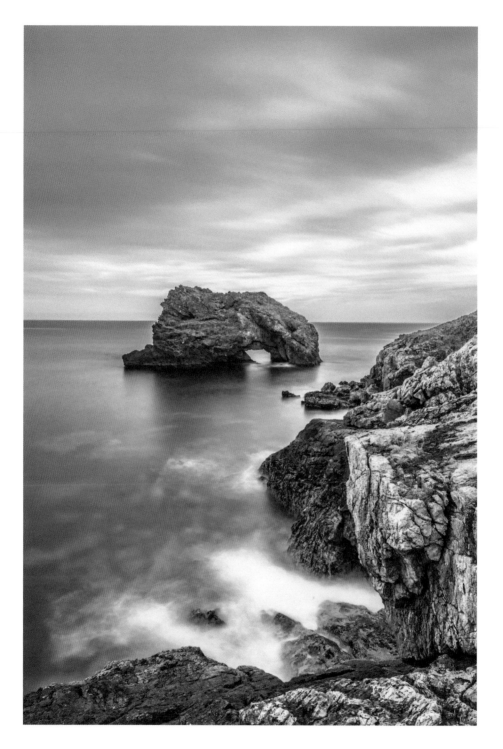

I've heard that the average distance a human can see to the horizon is around 3 miles, but I couldn't believe that to be true today.

The coastline seemed to be never ending, I could see for miles in every direction.

As I admired the view I heard the footsteps of somebody else climbing the stairs.
A woman entered the room, panting slightly, but smiling.

As we made small talk, the woman told me she had lived in the town her whole life.

The lighthouse was very important to her, she told me, because her grandfather had once lived there, as the lighthouse keeper. Fascinated, I listened as she told me more.

Her grandfather had been the lighthouse keeper for nearly 40 years. He had been a man of few words, but he was always very kind and helpful. He took great pride in keeping the lighthouse in good condition.

His job was to maintain the building, and repair any damages caused by the harsh coastal weather. And of course, to keep the light shining at night, to help guide sailors home.

Her grandfather had been a well respected man in the local community, known for his bravery and strength, and for his countless rescues of sailors in trouble at sea. He had braved dangerous storms and rough seas to save those who had been shipwrecked.

Hundreds of years ago lighthouses were lit by coal fires. It was a difficult and hard task to keep the flame alight, as lighthouse keepers would have to haul the coal to the top of the building and stoke the fire day and night.

Coal was eventually replaced by oil lamps, and by the end of the 18th century a rotating light had been developed using the same mechanisms that powered wristwatches.

I looked out at the ocean, quietly reflecting on what the lighthouse had meant to so many sailors, and to the families of this small seaside town.

It was a beacon of safety, and a reminder that even in the darkest of times, there is always hope.

Snorkelling

I walked back along the pier, my mind whirring with everything that I had learnt so far today. I felt so much more connected to this small town, with its rich history and kind locals.

I made my way back to the beach and arrived to find my family getting ready to go into the sea.

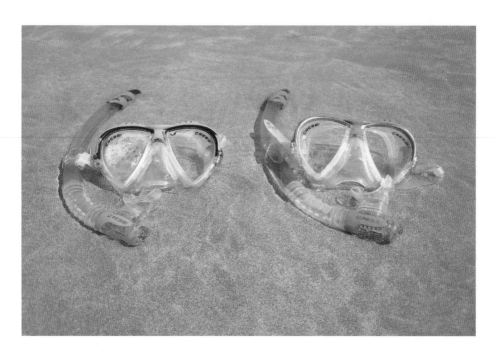

"Come join us, we're going to go snorkelling!"

Excitedly, I grabbed my goggles and snorkel and walked over to the sea with them. As we paddled into the water we laughed in surprise at how cold it was. It was wonderfully refreshing.

I put on my googles and snorkel, and gave a thumbs up to show that I was ready to go.

I began to slowly swim and looked down into the water. It was like looking into another world! The sunlight filtered through the gently swaying water to create a dappled glow on the sandy ocean floor.

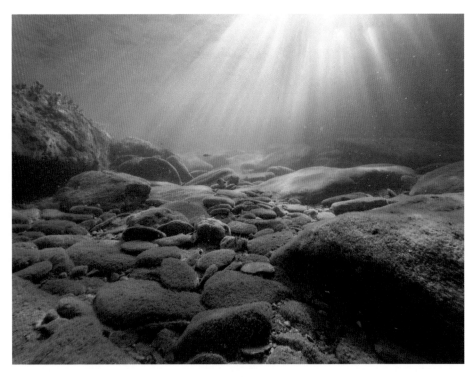

It was like swimming in a liquid rainbow, with flashes of blue, green and gold sparkling all around me.

Nestled within the sand were small rocks and stones. I picked one up.

It was particularly shiny this stone and it seemed to gleam like an emerald. In the flowing water it looked like a precious jewel, smooth and polished. A small treasure from the ocean.

I felt weightless and free, gliding through the water. It was so beautiful and serene, I felt like I was in a dream.

As I continued swimming I saw small fishes darting around, playing with each other.

I was so close I could see their tiny scales and bright eyes. They were so colourful, with their yellow, blue and green scales which glinted in the sunlight. I floated in the water and watched them, enjoying their beauty and playful nature.

I had read somewhere recently that it's estimated there are over 3 million shipwrecks scattered on the ocean floor across the world.

I wondered if I might find one today, covered in barnacles and coral.

How amazing it would be to find a large, lost sailing ship, resting on the sandy sea bed, filled with gold and treasure!

As I swam around exploring the ocean, I thought about how much fun a shipwreck must be for fish and other sea creatures. It would seem like an underwater skyscraper to them! So many spaces for the fish to explore and hide in.

After swimming around for a while, I decided today wasn't going to be my lucky day of finding a long, lost treasure ship. Alas!

I paddled out of the ocean with my family, laughing at how our fingers had pruned from the water.

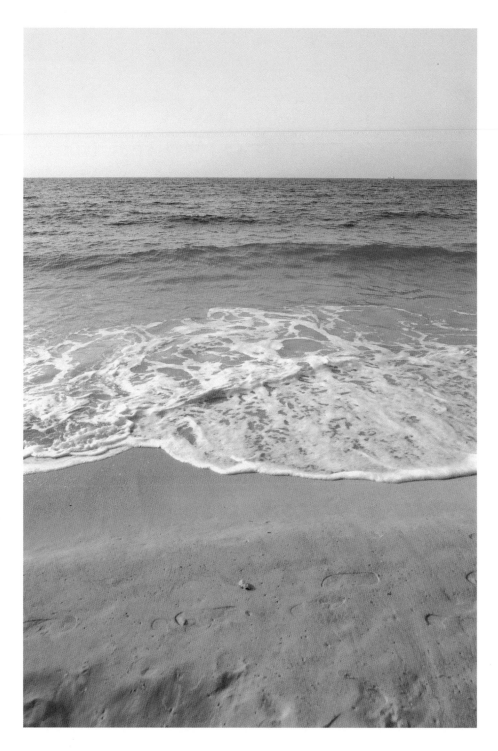

Walk Along The Promenade

As we dried the salty sea water off our skin we decided to take a walk together along the promenade. There was a light and pleasant breeze in the air. It was mid afternoon and the sun was still high in the sky.

Strolling along the wooden planks of the promenade we passed souvenir shops selling t-shirts, fridge magnets and coffee mugs.

Each shop seemed to have thousands of things on display, colourful knick knacks piled high and filling every space.

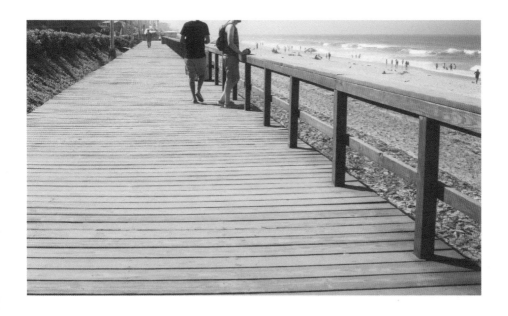

As we passed an arcade, the air was filled with the bright neon lights and sounds of the games.

The tinkling of coins being dropped into machines, the clanging and whirring of pinball machines, the screams of delight and laughter as players won games.

Although we were tempted to go into the arcade, we continued walking by, laughing as we saw a family pulling funny faces in a photo booth.

Continuing along the promenade we came to a large building. Peering inside through the windows, we could see an elegant ballroom. The room was beautifully decorated, with a large polished oak wooden floor.

Glittering chandeliers hung from a high ceiling, casting a bright golden glow on the room.

The room was filled with tables covered in white tablecloths, and a band played from a raised platform. It was a very grand space.

Couples were dancing together, gliding around and waltzing without a care in the world. We watched as they swayed to the music, moving with such beauty and grace. I have always loved dancing and watching others perform.

The term 'ballroom dancing' comes from the Latin word 'ballare' which means 'to dance'. My favourite dance has always been the Foxtrot, with its smooth and elegant steps.

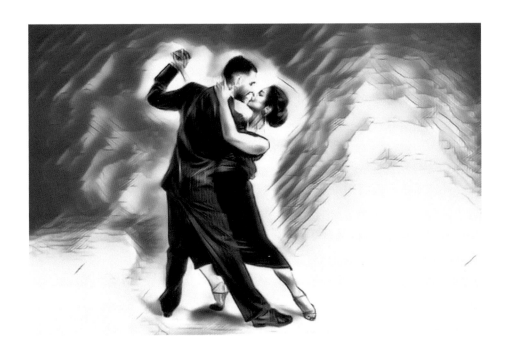

One couple in the ballroom seemed to be particularly good dancers.

The woman wore a flowing yellow dress, and the man was in a smart suit. They moved together in perfect harmony, as if they were gliding on air.

They spun and twirled around the room, dancing with such joy and passion, never taking their eyes off each other.

Pulling our eyes away from the window and marvelling at how good the dancers were, we began to wander back to the beach to enjoy the last few hours of sun together.

Golden Sunset

After shaking the sand off my towel, I lay down to enjoy the sunshine. The warmth of the sun felt wonderful on my skin. It was so relaxing, lying there, listening to the ebb and flow of the waves.

As I lay there, letting the world pass me by, I began to drift off to sleep, the sound of the ocean lulling me into a peaceful slumber.

I'm not sure how long I slept for, but when I woke the sun was beginning to lower in the sky. I felt wonderfully rested.

As I sat there, I watched the sun begin to set. The sky was filled with the most gorgeous display of colours.

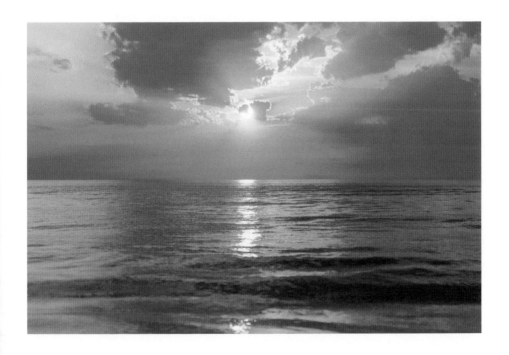

A warm golden glow spread across the sky, painting the clouds with shades of orange and pink. The ocean water sparkled and danced under the rays of sunlight.

As the sun sank lower in the sky, the beach grew quieter. Families were slowly packing up their things and heading home. But we decided to stick around and enjoy the sunset.

We enjoyed a nice, quiet moment together, peacefully taking in the last fleeting moments of the golden hour, as the sun bid farewell and tucked itself to sleep under the vast horizon.

The sea mirrored the colour of the sky and slowly transformed into a soft lilac glow.

As the sun dipped below the horizon and the light began to fade, we talked happily about what a wonderful day it had been. We slowly made our way back to the car, washing the sand off our feet when we reached the edge of the beach.

Exhausted but happy, we drove back home in the car. We knew we would return again one day, to create more wonderful memories together by the sea. We knew we would remember this special day forever.

Printed in Great Britain
by Amazon

26726503R00037